300
Incredible Things
for Health, Fitness & Diet
on the
Internet

300Incredible.com, LLC
600 Village Trace, Building 23
Marietta, Georgia 30067

(800) 909-6505

ISBN 0-9658668-7-4

Introduction

Here's to your health! This book will help you—through the Internet—find useful information about achieving and maintaining a healthy lifestyle. And if you seek details about specific diseases or illnesses, the sites in this book will efficiently guide you to the best resources. Be well.

Peter Lupus and Ken Leebow
Leebow@300INCREDIBLE.COM
http://www.300INCREDIBLE.COM

Notice

This book lists what we believe to be interesting and helpful health, fitness and diet sites on the Internet. We are not health professionals and are not qualified to and have not tried to determine the correctness or completeness of the information contained on these sites. Therefore, the sites included should be used for general educational purposes only, and each individual should consult with his or her own certified health professional for all specific advice related to health, fitness and diet.

About the Authors

Peter Lupus, best known for his role in the television series *Mission: Impossible,* is a recognized health, exercise and diet authority as well as an internationally known movie and television star. His association with celebrities all over the world has revealed to him the secrets of physically beautiful people, and his own outstanding physical appearance has earned him such titles as "Mr. Indiana" and "Mr. International Health."

In addition to acting and writing, Peter has served as professional consultant to the nation's top health spas and figure salons. He has been a frequent guest on many television shows, and his views on exercise and nutrition have generated a great demand for his guidance in personal health programs.

Ken Leebow has been in the computer business for over 20 years. The Internet has fascinated him since he began exploring its riches a few years ago, and he has helped thousands of individuals and businesses understand and utilize its resources. When not on the Net, you can find Ken playing tennis, running, reading or spending time with his family. He is living proof that being addicted to the Net doesn't mean giving up on the other pleasures of life.

Acknowledgments

Putting a book together requires many expressions of appreciation. We do this with great joy, as there are several people who have played vital roles in the process. We especially want to thank:

- Our families for being especially supportive during the writing of the book.

- Paul Joffe and Janet Bolton, of *TBI Creative Services*, for their editing and graphics skills.

- Mark Krasner and Janice Caselli for sharing our vision of the book and helping make it a reality.

- The multitude of great people who have encouraged and assisted us via e-mail.

Books by Ken Leebow

300 Incredible Things to Do on the Internet

300 Incredible Things for Kids on the Internet

300 Incredible Things for Sports Fans on the Internet

300 Incredible Things for Golfers on the Internet

300 Incredible Things for Travelers on the Internet

300 Incredible Things for Health, Fitness & Diet on the Internet

America Online Web Site Directory
Where to Go for What You Need

TABLE OF CONTENTS

TABLE OF CONTENTS (continued)

i

CHAPTER I
THE BEST OF HEALTH

1
Health on the Net

http://www.hon.ch
When you visit health sites on the Net, you will often see the HON logo. To earn this logo, the site must subscribe to the eight principles of credibility that HON developed.

2
My MD

http://www.personalmd.com
You deserve your own MD! This site has everything—a dictionary, encyclopedia, drug database, news and health centers. Best of all, you can personalize the site for your own needs.

3
WebMD

http://www.webmd.com
From current news to all of the major health topics, this MD has the information you need.

4
Adam and You

http://www.adam.com
Get your very own Personal Health Report. Find out: "How does my health compare to the average for my age and gender? What is my risk of heart disease or breast cancer? What can I do to reduce my risks?"

5
My Health

http://www.myhealtheon.com
All of the issues related to health are discussed here. You can also create your own health page and record your family's health data.

6
Patient's Health Guide
http://www3.bc.sympatico.ca/me/patientsguide
Here's a step-by-step guide to locating and researching medical conditions on the Internet.

7
MedLine
http://www.nlm.nih.gov/medlineplus
The National Library of Medicine offers a health directory and many dictionaries to assist with your health-related research.

8
Be Well
http://www.onhealth.com
News, articles, a reference section and an area that explains hundreds of ailments can be found here.

9
Dr. Johns

http://www.intelihealth.com
Hopkins, that is. Let this well-respected medical university assist with all your health needs.

10
Health Oasis

http://www.mayohealth.org
The world famous Mayo Clinic has current news, research centers ("allergies" to "women") and a library that has many interesting quizzes.

11
Medical Landscape

http://www.medscape.com
Medscape was designed for the medical professional. Now, this information is available to all.

12
It Takes a Village

http://www.betterhealth.com
The folks at IVillage.com offer a community-based Web site for better health.
Even if you don't join, you will be able to obtain valuable health information.

13
Portal to Health

http://www.healthwell.com
HealthWell's claim to fame is that it allows you to personalize its site for your
needs. Answer a few questions, and you'll have a Web site just for your health.

14
The Health Network

http://www.ahn.com
A mall, health tools, a section about conditions and diseases and much more
are provided.

15
Health Self Management

http://www.healthy.net

This site says, "We recognize that—more than any health professional, no matter how qualified or proficient—the individual is primarily responsible for his or her own health and well being." This site will assist with this responsibility.

16
May I Refer You?

http://www.medicinenet.com

Here's a group of doctors who strive to bring their perspective to important medical issues. Their goal is to be comprehensive and easy-to-use. You'll find news, facts, treatments and more.

17
Medical Help

http://medhlp.netusa.net
MedHelp is dedicated to helping patients find the highest quality medical information in the world today. They do this by offering a search engine, news and specific health topics.

18
Health Scout

http://www.healthscout.com
You'll find current news, a health directory, encyclopedias and much more.

19
Explore the Net

http://www.medexplorer.com
Medexplorer's tagline is "Your Health and Medical Center," and the site will guide you to valuable health information on the Net.

20
A to Z Health

http://www.healthatoz.com
You can search over 50,000 professionally reviewed health and medical
Internet resources. It even has a health organizer where you can track your
own health.

21
Thrive Online

http://www.thriveonline.com
ThriveOnline offers expert information, message board topics, chats,
interactive tools and information in six major areas: medical, fitness, nutrition,
serenity, sexuality and weight.

22
Get Healthy!

http://www.healthfinder.gov
At this site, the U.S. Department of Health and Human Services offers
reliable consumer health and human service information.

23
Oh Canada
http://www.hc-sc.gc.ca/english
This site says, "Here's to the good health of 30,850,000 Canadians," but there are lots of good resources for the entire world.

24
It's Your Health
http://www.yourhealth.com
http://www.yourhealth.com/ahl
Get information on a different health topic every week. One of the most interesting areas is the audio health library (AHL).

25
Bless You
http://www.achoo.com
This Web portal has tons of great health information. Use the search engine, the site of the week and the archives to find great information.

26
Get Physical…

http://www.phys.com

…with the folks from Conde Nast. Major categories include fitness, nutrition, weight loss and pregnancy.

27
Healthy Answers

http://www.healthanswers.com

This site wants to be your sole source for health information. It has health centers for topics ranging from addiction to women's health. Go here for a checkup today.

28
Stay Well

http://www.wellweb.com

From A to Z, you'll find almost every subject area covered at the patient's network. Check out the master index for details.

29
You First

http://www.youfirst.com

Take care of yourself! Start by taking the Health Risk Assessment test. You'll get recommendations about improving your health and minimizing potential future health problems.

30
Grade A

http://www.healthgrades.com

This site gives grades and offers advice on finding physicians, hospitals and health plans.

31
50 Something

http://www.thirdage.com

Third Age is a site that addresses the needs and concerns of the baby boom generation. If that's you, this might be a good place for you to hang out.

32
It's Your Choice

http://www.healthychoice.com
The Healthy Choice food company offers a great site that has news, recipes, fitness tips and many links to visit.

33
California Dreaming

http://www.mylifepath.com
Blue Shield of California has a health and wellness site for all. It has cool tools and covers just about every health topic.

34
Health Profile

http://www.healthcentral.com
Get a free health profile at HealthCentral.

35
Medical Terminology

http://www3.bc.sympatico.ca/me/patientsguide/medterms.htm
http://www3.bc.sympatico.ca/me/patientsguide/glossary.htm
Medical terms can often be a little bewildering. Here are your online medical term dictionaries.

36
Mental Help

http://mentalhelp.net
http://www.mentalhealth.org/links/KENLINKS.htm
Here are mental health directories and guides.

37
Organize This

http://www.ktv-i.com/helpagen/by_name.cfm
http://www.wtvc.com/medlinks.html
There are many organizations and associations that can assist with various medical issues. Here is a list of many of them.

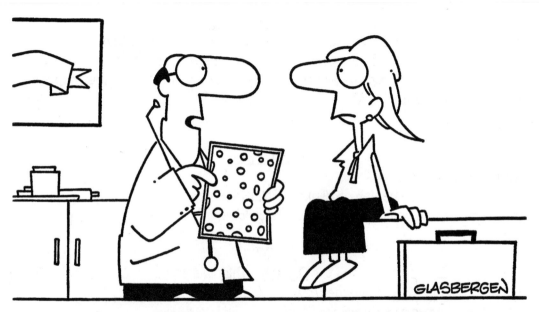

"The red blobs are your red blood cells.
The white blobs are your white blood cells.
The brown blobs are coffee. We need to talk."

38
Pearly Whites
http://www.ada.org/tc-cons.html
This is the American Dental Association patient site. All types of dental care and issues are discussed, and there are different sections for parents, kids, adults and seniors.

39
Health and Minorities
http://raceandhealth.hhs.gov
The U.S. is committed to eliminating the disparities in six areas of health status experienced by racial and ethnic minority populations, while continuing the progress made in improving the overall health of the American people.

40
Medical Privacy
http://washofc.epic.org/privacy/medical
Be aware of medical privacy issues. "Whatsoever things I see or hear concerning the life of men, in my attendance on the sick or even apart therefrom, which ought not be noised abroad, I will keep silence thereon, counting such things to be as sacred secrets."—from the Oath of Hippocrates, 4th Century, B.C.E.

41
Get Well Soon
http://www.bluemountainarts.com
Do you know someone who needs a little cheering up? Send an e-mail get well card. It's thoughtful, quick and free.

CHAPTER II
GET FIT

42
Shape Up!

http://www.shapeup.org
Shape Up America is a national initiative to promote healthy weight and increased physical activity in America.

43
Just Move It!

http://www.justmove.org
The American Heart Association offers this Fitness Center that has an exercise diary, fitness news and fitness comparison charts.

44
Sleep Well
http://www.stanford.edu/~dement
We often take sleep for granted, but if you have any problems sleeping, this is a site for sore eyes.

45
Stretch with Carol
http://www.stretch.com
Learn all types of stretches that can be done almost anywhere.

46
Get Active
http://chitrib.webpoint.com/fitness
The Chicago Tribune provides this simple and elegant Web site that offers much information about fitness.

47
Know Thy Body

http://www.innerbody.com
Use this site to learn the basics about your body.

48
Muscle Groups

http://www.global-fitness.com/strength/s_map.html
Just click on a muscle group, and you'll receive an explanation and exercise instruction for strength training that part of the body.

49
Bodies in Motion…Minds at Rest

http://library.advanced.org/12153
It states at this site: "Improve your health, both physically and mentally. Learn what you can do to get in good shape and stay that way. Learn how to better yourself as a person and be a good companion. Learn how to deal with the issues that affect you."

50
E-Card for Fitness
http://www.americanheart.org/ecard
Send an electronic fitness greeting card to help inspire one of your loved ones.

51
All the News That's Fit
http://www.fitnesslink.com
From news to links, you'll find it here.

52
Fitness Partner
http://primusweb.com/fitnesspartner
Partners help us stay motivated. On the Net, the Fitness Partner does that.

53
Yoga.com

http://www.yogaclass.com
http://www.yogasite.com
The health benefits of Yoga have been documented for centuries, and these sites will give you the details.

54
Feel Great, Look Great

http://www.ivillage.com/fitness
That's the philosophy at this site. You'll find tips, experts, calculators and other tools to assist with your fitness program.

55
Open for Fitness

http://www.24hourfitness.com
Here are tips and information about fitness, nutrition, health…and you can ask Dr. Steele any fitness question.

56
A World of Fitness

http://www.worldfitness.org
There's a world of straightforward and honest information at this site.

57
Online Fitness

http://www.fitnessonline.com
Exercise, nutrition, mind and body are all covered here. If you want your own personalized page, just answer a few questions.

58
No Stress

http://www.teachhealth.com
Got stress in your life? Let Dr. Burns assist you in this area. He does it in a fun and easy-to-read format.

59
Pumping Iron
http://www.cyberpump.com
News, training tips, a Q&A section and more are featured. Get pumped up.

60
Weightlifting is Us
http://www.weightsnet.com
WeightsNet is a resource for people who work out with weights for bodybuilding, fitness, powerlifting, sports and more.

61
Strongman
http://www.seriousfun.net/weightlifting/categories.htm
You'll find information relating to bodybuilding, powerlifting and Olympic-style weightlifting at this site.

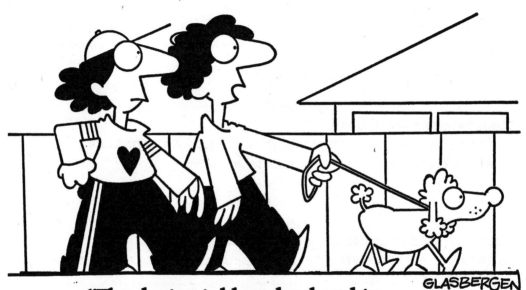

"The doctor told my husband to double his physical activity, so now he changes channels with both hands."

62
Muscle & Fitness
http://www.muscle-fitness.com
This is for everyone that has or desires to have a hard body.

63
Athletic Conditioning
http://www.completeconditioning.com
You'll find many fine articles and other interesting items at this site.

64
Fit for Business
http://www.fitforbusiness.com
Fit For Business gives you all of the information you need to maintain your health and productivity on the road.

65
Runners Take Your Mark

http://www.kicksports.com

This is a complete online resource for runners—a one-stop reference guide on all aspects of training, racing, nutrition and running gear.

66
Everyone's Running

http://www.runnersworld.com

Running continues to be one of the most popular fitness routines, and Runner's World is here for support. Check out the Health and Fitness section.

CHAPTER III
EAT TO LIVE

67
Pyramid Power
http://www.nal.usda.gov:8001/py/pmap.htm
No need to go to Egypt, this pyramid is a guide to your daily food choices.

68
What's in a Label?
http://www.fda.gov/opacom/backgrounders/foodlabel/newlabel.html
Food labels got you confused? Check this site out, and you will become a knowledgeable food label reader.

69
Focus on Nutrition
http://www.nutritionnewsfocus.com
http://www.nutrition4you.com
Take charge of your own nutrition. Review articles, ask experts and receive a daily e-mail newsletter.

70
The FDA
http://www.fda.gov
http://www.foodsafety.gov
Check out what the Food and Drug Administration is doing for you. And while you're at it, go to the government's gateway for food safety.

71
A Ton o' Links
http://www.arborcom.com
The Arbor Guide has information about nutrition, alternative medicine, food science and more. Stay here for a while and check out the "Land of Links."

72
Eat Well, Live Well

http://www.healthyeating.org
Online surveys, checklists, articles and sections for professionals, the general public, students and kids can be found at this site from Down Under.

73
Fruits and Veggies

http://www.5aday.gov
http://www.dole5aday.com
http://dccps.nci.nih.gov/5aday
The National 5 A Day for Better Health Program gives Americans a simple, positive message: "Eat 5 or more servings of fruits and vegetables every day for better health."

74
Healthy Refrigerator
http://www.healthyfridge.org
A healthy home starts with a healthy refrigerator. Open this cool, entertaining and informative site. And for football fans, there is a "calm" Coach Ditka featured.

75
Educate the Masses
http://www.cspinet.org
The Center for Science in the Public Interest seeks to promote health through educating the public about nutrition and alcohol.

76
The Blonz Guide
http://www.blonz.com
Dr. Ed has a guide to nutrition on the Net. He has written many books about the subject.

77
Nutrition Navigator
http://navigator.tufts.edu
Tuft's University rates nutrition sites on the Net. This site gets an A+.

78
IFICF
http://ificinfo.health.org
The International Food Information Council Foundation provides consumers and educators with tips for food safety and nutrition.

79
Fruits and Veggies
http://www.produceoasis.com
Get tips, recipes and detailed information about fruits and vegetables.

80
Nutritional Analysis

http://www.ag.uiuc.edu/~food-lab/nat/mainnat.html
http://cgi.fatfree.com/cgi-bin/fatfree/usda/usda.cgi
Type in a food item, and get a complete nutritional analysis.

81
Nutrition Action

http://www.cspinet.org/nah
Here are tips and some great articles about nutrition.

82
You Are What You Eat

http://library.advanced.org/11163
In conjunction with a program called ThinkQuest, students have developed
this interesting and informative site about nutrition.

83
Open the Fridge
http://www.familyfoodzone.com
Have fun with this refrigerator, and learn a lot about your food.

84
Sports Nutrition
http://www.sportsparents.com/nutrition/index.html
Sports Illustrated for Kids has an area dedicated to sports nutrition.

85
Delicious Decisions
http://www.deliciousdecisions.org
The American Heart Association will show you how "delicious" and "nutritious" can have everything in common.

86
Nutrition and Food on the Web
http://www.sfu.ca/~jfremont

Jean Fremont has a fun page called: "Finding the Right Stuff." No doubt, you'll find interesting Web sites and articles to assist with your nutritional needs and knowledge.

87
Read the Label
http://vm.cfsan.fda.gov/label.html

Every food product has a label describing the food content. Do you read it? Learn all about the labeling at the Food and Drug Administration's site.

88
Body Mass Index
http://www.nhlbisupport.com/bmi

What's yours? Provide your height and weight, and you'll instantly know.

89
Eat Right!

http://www.writeeating.com
Gisele Guilbert Anderson is your "Write Eating" coach. Use her Web site and rational approach to eating.

90
Favorite Conversation

http://www.diettalk.com
Diettalk is a directory of good diet information. Start with the calculator section, and proceed from there.

91
Diet Analysis

http://dawp.anet.com
At this site, enter the foods you've eaten for one day and receive a complete nutritional review of your diet based on the Recommended Dietary Allowances for your demographic profile.

92
It's Your Body

http://www.bodyisland.com
Take care of it with BodyIsland. This site has live chats, news, a weekly issues section and many tips.

93
The Hacker's Diet

http://www.fourmilab.ch/hackdiet
Here's an interesting and unique diet book—online. The premise is an engineer businessman who decided that being fat was a problem to be solved, not a burden to be endured.

94
For Weight Loss

http://www.4weightloss.com
It seems like everyone wants to lose weight. Here's a directory that can help.

95
Watch Your Weight

http://www.dietwatch.com
Here's an Internet support group for watching your weight. Come for a visit and a tour.

96
What's Your Goal?

http://www.dietsite.com
This site will help you choose healthy foods when dining, get diet advice and obtain up-to-date and straightforward nutrition information.

97
Calorie Conscious

http://www.caloriecontrol.org
This site says, "If you're looking for information on cutting calories and fat in your diet, achieving and maintaining a healthy weight, or your favorite low-calorie, reduced-fat foods, then you've come to the right place!"

98
Ask the Dietitian
http://www.dietitian.com
People have asked questions about everything from alcohol to zinc, and this site has the answers.

99
Cyberdiet
http://www.cyberdiet.com
If you want to adopt a healthy lifestyle, Cyberdiet is here for support.

100
American Dietetic Association
http://www.eatright.org
The ADA offers tips, featured articles, nutrition resources and more.

101
National Cholesterol Education
http://rover.nhlbi.nih.gov/chd
We're always hearing about cholesterol, and now you can learn more from the National Institutes of Health.

102
Low Fat Recipes
http://www.gourmetspot.com/lowfatrecipes.htm
This site will take you to many fine, low fat recipe sites.

103
Fast Food Calculator
http://www.olen.com/food
Learn the nutritional information for more than 1,000 fast-food items.

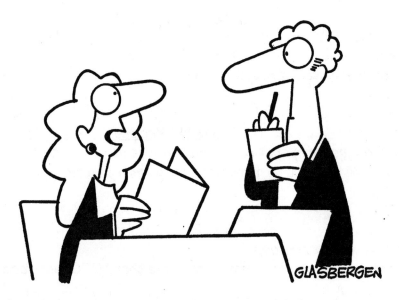

"I'm going to order a broiled skinless chicken breast, but I want you to bring me lasagna and garlic bread by mistake."

104
Food Terminology
http://ificinfo.health.org/glossary.htm
Here's a food glossary for you. We hear many of these terms every day, and now you have a place to get quick definitions.

105
The Millennium
http://www.weightloss2000.com
What's your resolution for the new millennium? To lose weight? Let the resources of Weightloss2000 assist.

106
Name Brand Diets

http://www.weightwatchers.com
http://www.jennycraig.com
http://www.zoneperfect.com
http://www.atkinsdiet.com
http://www.richardsimmons.com
http://www.sugarbusters.com

Have you tried any of these popular weight control programs and strategies?

CHAPTER IV
EXPERT ADVICE

107
Doctors Cry, Too
http://www.dr-boehm.com
Dr. Boehm has written many essays. Sit back, relax and read the interesting writings of this thoughtful doctor.

108
Family Doc
http://www.familydoctor.org
You'll find topics and issues for men, women, children and seniors. There are sections with detailed information on the body and common conditions.

109
Dr. Quackwatch

http://www.quackwatch.com

Dr. Stephen Barrett calls this site "Your Guide to Health Fraud, Quackery and Intelligent Decisions."

110
Debunk Junk

http://www.junkscience.com

Steve Milloy refers to this subject matter as "all the junk that's fit to debunk." While this site is not only about health, many of the issues that are addressed are related to health and medicine.

111
Real Doctors

http://www.americasdoctor.com

Real doctors, real answers, real time, 24 hours a day. Chat with a doctor, join a community or read timely articles.

112
What's Up Doc?

http://www.docguide.com
This doc will guide you to information and sites that are intended to assist doctors and patients.

113
American Family Physician

http://www.aafp.org/afp/patient.html
The American Academy of Family Physicians offers a patient section that addresses many health issues. Scan the site and see if you need information on any of these topics.

114
Better Health...

http://www.netwellness.org
...through information. Three major universities in Ohio have joined to create this site. You can ask questions and research all health topics.

115
Celebrity Doctors

http://www.drruth.com
http://www.drlaura.com
http://www.drweil.com
http://www.drkoop.com
http://www.randomhouse.com/seussville
Dr. Sex, Dr. Feel Good, Dr. Alternative, Dr. Former Surgeon General and maybe the one who brings the most joy to your heart—Dr. Seuss.

116
Deepak

http://www.chopra.com
From the comfort of your computer, learn the essence of Deepak on the Net. "We directly experience the expansion of our consciousness as we connect with each other in our shared quest for greater knowledge."

117
Surgeon General
http://www.surgeongeneral.gov
Since 1871, the Surgeon General of the United States has been the nation's leading spokesman on matters of public health. Meet the current Surgeon General—Dr. David Satcher.

118
On Call Docs
http://www.thehealthchannel.com/oncall
There are also many less famous doctors online who can help

119
Celeb Situations
http://www.adoctorinyourhouse.com
Stephanie Powers profiles some well-known figures and their health issues.

120
Life's Challenges

http://www.drbernie.com
Dr. Bernie provides a guide for living life's challenges.

121
Family Health

http://www.rosemond.com
Let John Rosemond come into your home or office (through the Net) and provide practical and simple advice for reducing the stress of your family life.

122
Doctor's Rag

http://www.physweekly.com
Read the magazine that doctors read. There are some very interesting articles at this site.

123
Find a Doc

http://www.thelittlebluebook.com
http://www.doctordirectory.com
These sites allow you to search for a doctor online.

124
Board Certified

http://certifieddoctor.org/verify.html
It seems that many people are hesitant to ask if their doctors are board certified or not. Go to this site and find out.

125
Doctors On Call

http://www.doctorsoncall.com
Doctors On Call (DOC) is the largest medical professional directory on the Web. Search from a list of 400,000 U.S. doctors.

126
What's Up Doc?

http://www.locateadoc.com
At this site, you can search for a doctor or ask a question of an entire panel of doctors.

127
How Much?

http://www.napr.org
http://www.pohly.com/salary.shtml
Many people are obsessed with how much money doctors make. Check out salaries here.

128
First Aid

http://firstaid.ie.eu.org
This site states, "The life you save may be the life you love." Learn first aid techniques for many types of occurrences.

129
Active First Aid Book
http://www.parasolemt.com.au/afa
This is an online first aid book written by ambulance paramedics with a total of 40 years experience in pre-hospital care.

130
Expert Advice
http://www.askanexpert.com
Choose an expert in one of the categories, and you will be well on your way to finding a solution.

131
Stanford's Healthlink
http://www-med.stanford.edu/healthlink
This fine institution provides a health tip each and every day, plus health radio, news and links.

132
Go Ask Alice

http://www.goaskalice.columbia.edu
Alice answers questions on many health-related issues. She has answered so
many questions at the Web site, that she now also has a book.

133
Daily Tip

http://www.cybertip4theday.com
Receive a daily tip from the health-related category of your choice.

134
Travel Health

http://www.drwisetravel.com
If your health is an issue when traveling, this doctor might be able to assist.

135
Insurance Assistance

http://www.life-line.org
Get straightforward and unbiased information on insurance—life, health and disability.

136
The Eyes Have It

http://www.opticaladvisor.com
At the Optical Advisor, you can explore eyeglasses, lenses, frames, contact lenses and other vision care issues. Ironically, not all of the information is immediately visible, so make sure you click on a few buttons. If you do, you'll find a glossary and more.

137
Tips and Tools
http://www.healthcalc.net
http://www.heartinfo.com
Get a tip a day. Answer a few questions, and you can also get your target heart rate, body mass index, energy expenditure and some interesting basic nutritional information.

138
Why?
http://whyfiles.news.wisc.edu/oldstorylist.html
Got a health question? The Whyfiles may have the answer.

139
Learn About Health
http://www.learn2.com/browse/hea.html
The folks from Learn2.com will teach you about many different health-related topics—for example, "learn to stretch."

140
Can We Chat?

http://www.healthguide.com
The Health Guide has many areas of health — body, mind, cancer, family, pharmacy, professional, seniors and wellness. In addition to the detailed information, you can send messages to other people on the Net.

141
Healthy Conversations

http://www.deja.com
"Share what you know, and learn what you don't." People on the Net are happy to share their knowledge. If you have a question or a solution, get involved at this site.

142
Mail Health

http://www.liszt.com
Become a part of the e-mail revolution, and join a health-related e-mail discussion list.

143
Can We Talk?

http://www.healthboards.com
From acne to women's health, this site has message boards for you to converse with your fellow Netizens.

144
Let's Chat

http://www.yack.com
http://www.talkcity.com
http://chat.yahoo.com
Just click on "health," and you will be propelled into the world of chat rooms for that subject area. Talking with other folks about your issues will often achieve positive results.

145
Support Me
http://www.support-group.com
Support-Group.com allows people with health, personal, and relationship issues to share their experiences through Bulletin Boards and Online Chat. It also has links to support-related information on the Internet.

146
I've Got A Headache
http://www.excedrin.com
In addition to promoting Excedrin products, this site is a major resource specializing in information about headache problems.

147
Alternative Opinions
http://www.juiceguy.com/healthinfo
This page is intended to provide alternative opinions to conventional wisdom on health. Even if you don't agree with all it says, it is still very entertaining.

148
Be Natural

http://www.naturalland.com

You'll find all types of interesting and fun things here—quizzes, community groups and news by different health categories.

149
Herbs Galore

http://www.botanical.com

Here's a hypertext version of "A Modern Herbal." This huge book contains over 800 varieties of medicinal, culinary and cosmetic herbs, including economic properties, cultivation and folklore. You'll also find many interesting links.

150
The Nobel Prize

http://www.nobel.se/prize/index.html

See the winners of the Nobel Prize in medicine since 1901.

CHAPTER V
AILMENTS AND TREATMENTS

151
Smoke Free

http://www.tobaccofreekids.org
http://just.about.com/quitsmoking
http://www.quitsmokingsupport.com
Here's the Campaign for Tobacco-Free Kids. Let's face it, if you never start, you'll be a lot healthier. And if by chance you are still smoking, check out these sites that will help you quit.

152
Center for Disease Control

http://www.cdc.gov
The CDC has sections for men's, women's, and seniors' health. You'll also find a Health A–Z section that discusses most of the major diseases.

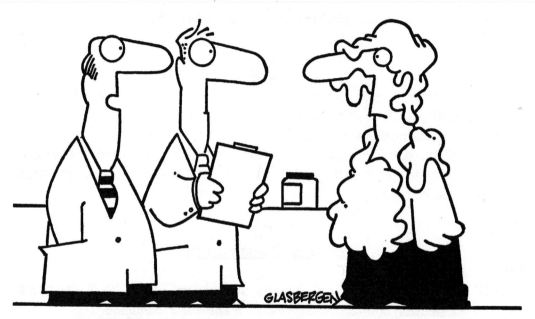

"With this new drug, cholesterol forms *outside* of the body, where it can't clog the arteries."

153
Well Healed

http://www.healingwell.com
HealingWell is a guide to diseases, disorders and chronic illness. Pick a
category, and you will find message boards, online resources and much more.

154
I'm Addicted

http://www.well.com/user/woa/index.html
http://www.hubplace.com/addictions
http://www.alcoholismhelp.com
If you have an addiction or know someone else who does, this might be a good
starting point to obtain information.

155
Pain Relief

http://www.pain.com
http://www.aapainmanage.org
These sites contain pain information for the professional and consumer. You'll find resources, chat rooms, news, articles and much more.

156
All Allergies

http://www.allergy.pair.com
If you are an allergy sufferer, these sites are for you. You'll find helpful articles, books, databases and more.

157
Food Alert

http://www.foodallergy.org
This site has tips, product alerts, a newsletter and a section that separates fact from fiction.

158
American Heart Association
http://www.americanheart.org
This site proclaims to be "dedicated to providing you with education and information on fighting heart disease and stroke."

159
Heart Milestones
http://www.ahfmr.ab.ca/Jan1997/milestone.html
Make a quick visit here to learn about many of the milestones concerning the human heart.

160
Heart Guard
http://www.ahfmr.ab.ca/Jan1997/cartoon.html
http://www.glasbergen.com/fit.html
If you agree that laughter can be the best medicine, go to these cartoon sites for a dose or two.

161
American Lung Association
http://www.lungusa.org
Lung disease is the number three killer in America, responsible for one in seven deaths. This site has an amazing amount of information. Read the "Wall of Remembrance." It may have an impact on you or on someone you love.

162
NHLBI
http://www.nhlbi.nih.gov
The National Heart, Lung and Blood Institute (NHLBI) will provide you with information about research and educational activities. They will even tell you how to achieve your healthy weight.

163
Brain Tumor Association
http://www.abta.org
Research, information and resources are available to you—if you need them—at this association's site.

164
American Cancer Society

http://www.cancer.org

Prevention and early detection are two of the most important and effective strategies for reaching the American Cancer Society's goals of saving lives lost from cancer, diminishing suffering due to cancer and eliminating cancer as a major health problem.

165
Cancer Institute

http://cancernet.nci.nih.gov

http://www.cdc.gov/cancer/linksalt.htm

Unfortunately, we all know someone who has had cancer. These and other credible resources are needed when the disease hits someone close to us.

166
Beat It!

http://www.cancersurvival.org
This site will provide you with helpful information, including suggestions for increasing survival odds, recommended reading and useful links to important cancer sites on the Internet.

167
Prostate Cancer

http://www.prostateinfocenter.com
http://www.prostatecancer.on.ca
http://www.comed.com/Prostate
These sites are dedicated to "fighting for the 1 in 8 men (and their families) who will develop prostate cancer."

168
Confronting Cancer Through Art
http://www.oncolink.upenn.edu/ccta/full.html
http://www.oncolink.upenn.edu
Confronting Cancer Through Art is a unique exhibition that gives vision and voice to the experiences of those who have confronted cancer.

169
American Diabetes Association
http://www.diabetes.org
http://www.diabetesmonitor.com
The mission is "to prevent and cure diabetes and to improve the lives of all people affected by diabetes."

170
Children's Diabetes
http://www.wishcure.com
http://www.childrenwithdiabetes.com
Discover the online community for families who have a child with diabetes.

171
AIDS/HIV

http://www.aegis.com
http://www.thebody.com
These comprehensive sites will assist anyone who needs information about AIDS and HIV.

172
Alzheimer's

http://www.alz.org
http://www.alzforum.org
http://www.zarcrom.com/users/yeartorem
You'll find topics that include: "just the facts," "taking care," "medical issues," "research" and more.

173
Clinical Trials

http://www.centerwatch.com
Clinical trials, studies, research and new therapies can be found here.

174
Hospice

http://www.nho.org
When in need, this outstanding organization is there for us. Hospice care is a compassionate method of caring for terminally ill people.

175
Death with Dignity

http://www.growthhouse.org
Unfortunately, no matter what age we are now, we will all have to address this issue at some point. This site will assist in identifying helpful resources.

176
Alternative Medicine

http://www.alternativemedicine.com
Here's a large database of alternative medical information with the goals of helping you get well and stay well.

177
Another Opinion
http://www.altmedicine.com
You might want a second opinion when it comes to health care, so here's another excellent source for alternative medicine.

178
Spirituality and Health
http://www.spiritualityhealth.com
Ideas, advice, tests, news and other spiritual information are here for you. Come on in and learn more about your inner landscape.

179
A Healing Place in Cyberspace
http://www.journeyofhearts.org
This is "a Web site for anyone who has ever experienced a loss; a place for enhancing physical and mental well-being."

180
Acupuncture

http://www.acupuncture.com
What is acupuncture? Can it cure you? Where can you find an acupuncturist?
You'll find answers to all your questions here.

181
Don't Mess With Mother Nature

http://www.mothernature.com
While this site wants to sell you products, you can also find an interesting
encyclopedia, news and other information.

CHAPTER VI
TAKE YOUR MEDICINE

182
Drug Companies
http://www.druginfonet.com/maninfo.htm
Who are the drug manufacturers of the world? Find out here.

183
RxList
http://www.rxlist.com
http://www.virtualdrugstore.com
Is this your online pharmacist? No, but you can get a lot of information about various medications.

184
Drug Information

http://www.pharminfo.com
This is a great resource for news, articles and details about a lot of
prescription drugs.

185
Drugstores on the Net

http://cnn.com/HEALTH/9906/22/online.rx
http://www.ftc.gov/opa/1999/9907/pharma.htm
http://cnn.com/TECH/computing/9906/04/edrugs.idg
Is selling medications via the Internet ready for prime time? Though many
companies are already selling vitamins and prescription drugs on the Net, it is
important to be a careful and informed consumer.

186
Ye Old Internet Drugstore

http://www.drugstore.com
http://www.planetrx.com
Can't make it to your local pharmacy today? Well, now they'll come to you.

187
Offline and Online Drugstores

http://www.riteaid.com
http://www.cvs.com
http://www.walgreens.com
http://e-pharmacy-dev.cks.com
http://www.drugemporium.com
Some of your favorite offline drugstores have now begun to join the world of online e-commerce.

188
Top 200

http://www.drugtopics.com/brand.html
http://www.drugtopics.com/generic.html
Want to know the top 200 brand name and generic drugs? Make a stop here and you'll know.

189
Vitamin Advice

http://cgi.pathfinder.com/drweil/vitaminprofiler
Let the good doctor advise you as to which vitamins you should be taking.

190
Health Advice

http://www.vitamins.com
Its slogan is "lowest price or free." In addition to selling products, it offers free advice on all health issues—just like your trusted local pharmacist.

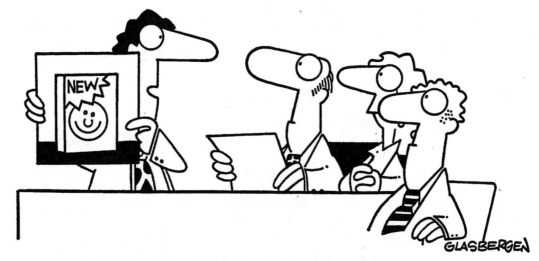

"Our new product has no fat, no cholesterol, no calories, no sugar, no salt and no preservatives. The box is empty, but it has exactly what everyone wants!"

191
E-Health and Nutrition

http://www.enutrition.com
You'll find articles and products about health, weight, fitness, nutrition and more at this site.

192
What's the Buzz?

http://www.vitaminbuzz.com
http://www.vitaminshoppe.com
Need to know more about vitamins? You can learn and buy here.

CHAPTER VII
AGE AND GENDER

193
Health Discovery
http://www.discoveryhealth.com
His, hers, kids, seniors and more—you'll discover it here.

194
Virtual Medical Center
http://www.mediconsult.com
Women, men and seniors—there's something here for everyone in these categories.

195
Having My Baby
http://www.babycenter.com
From preconception to toddler, the baby center will assist you.

196
Infant Nutrition
http://www.msnbc.com/news/295061.asp
Here's an article that presents seven steps to better infant nutrition.

197
Start 'em Young
http://www.bennygoodsport.com
You may as well learn about health at an early age. Benny is a good sport and takes the time to assist the little ones in the family.

198
Kids and Food
http://www.kidsfood.org
Kids, teachers and parents can all come to the food tree house to learn and have fun with food.

199
Pediatric Resource
http://www.pedinfo.org
Any area a pediatrician might address is at this Web site.

200
Pediatrics for Parents
http://www.momsrefuge.com/pediatrics
Each month, Dr. Rich Sagall, board certified Family Practitioner and Professor at Allegheny University of the Health Sciences, brings you the latest news in children's health.

201
Health for the Young
http://www.parentsplace.com/health
Most issues related to childcare are discussed here. Check out the "favorite tools" section and track your child's immunization records online.

202
Health and Safety in Child Care
http://nrc.uchsc.edu
All types of health and safety care issues for youngsters are discussed.

203
Kid's Health
http://www.kidshealth.org
KidsHealth has information on infections, behavior and emotions, food and fitness and growing up healthy. There are also games and animations.

204
ParentTime Health
http://www.pathfinder.com/ParentTime/Health/home/health.all.html
ParentTime is Time Warner's online parenting publication. This section is dedicated to health issues from infant to school age.

205
Souped Up Advice
http://www.parentsoup.com/library/hospital/index.html
Some of the concerns that all parents face are addressed at ParentSoup.

206
Drug Education
http://www.acde.org
The American Council for Drug Education has an informative, fact-filled site about drugs.

207
Attention Deficit Hyperactivity Disorder
http://www.nimh.nih.gov/publicat/adhd.htm
http://www.med.nyu.edu/Psych/addc/addscr.htm
http://www.chadd.org
http://www.addult.org
Attention Deficit Disorder has been receiving a lot of publicity. Study and learn about it at these sites.

208
Healthy Relationship

http://relationshipweb.com
Here's first aid for relationships, with a directory of thousands of helpful relationship links, discussion forums and more. No doubt, a healthy relationship can lead to a happy and less stressful life.

209
Enjoy Your Visit

http://www.gyn101.com
Most experts agree that females who are over 18 years old, or are sexually active, should have a gynecological exam every year. For background information, visit here first.

210
Take the Test

http://www.wdxcyber.com/test.htm
Ladies, how much do you know about your health? Take a test here to find out.

211
Having My Baby

http://www.epregnancy.com
http://www.pregnancycalendar.com
If it has to do with pregnancy, you will find it at these two wonderful sites.
Congratulations!

212
Choose Your Department

http://www.homearts.com/depts/health/00dphec1.htm
Natural Healing, the Body Beautiful, Breast Health, the Whole Nine Months, and Care Guide can be found here.

213
Healthy Women

http://www.womens-health.com
Health issues for the woman in mid-life are covered here. If you like big words, this site uses a lot of them.

214
For Women Only

http://www.women.com

Fitness, food and health are some of the categories at this super site. You can even create your own personalized page.

215
American Health

http://www.americanhealth.com

This magazine addresses good health for women. It has magazine articles online from 1996 to its current issue.

216
Women's Health

http://www.womenshealth.org

From beauty to sports and fitness, this site is a forum for women's health.

217
For the She in Us
http://www.herhealth.com
This site offers a holistic approach to general health, fitness, food and nutrition, mind and spirit, natural woman and sexuality.

218
Hot Flash
http://www.dearest.com/intro.htm
Everything you need to know about menopause is provided through this supportive community.

219
About Women's Health
http://womenshealth.about.com
Many of the health issues that women face are discussed here.

220
Women's Health Stories
http://cnn.com/HEALTH/womens.health/index.html
CNN and WebMD have current stories about issues of the day for women.

221
New York Times
http://www.nytimes.com/specials/women/whome/index.html
http://www.nytimes.com/specials/women/nyt98
The Times has articles and information especially for women. Make sure you check out the resource section.

222
Breast Cancer
http://www.cancerhelp.com
http://www.nationalbreastcancer.org
Find detailed information and quick links to the latest news in breast cancer research, prevention and treatment.

223
Male Health Center

http://www.malehealthcenter.com

This site has everything you ever wanted to know about health issues for men, but may have been afraid to ask.

224
AARP

http://www.aarp.org/healthguide/home.html

You don't have to be over fifty to take advantage of this site.

225
What is Medicare?

http://www.medicare.gov

At the official U.S. government site for Medicare information, you'll find out.

226
Respect Your Elders

http://www.elderweb.com
Elderweb has over 4,500 links to eldercare. Also featured is long-term care information on legal, financial, medical and housing issues, as well as policy, research and statistics.

227
Long-Term Care

http://www.mr-longtermcare.com
The following testimonial about this site says it best: "I want to thank Mr. Long-term Care for his commitment to improving long-term care and to educating the public about the great need for affordable quality care in this country." — Hillary Rodham Clinton.

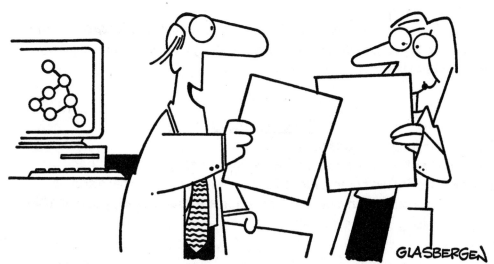

"Our new synthetic fat substitute is made entirely from wool. With our product, dieters will shrink when they get wet!"

228
Advice and Chat

http://www.seniors-site.com
This site has message boards and some people who may be able to answer your questions.

229
Government Assistance

http://www.seniors.gov/health.html
The U.S. government lists some of its Web sites that offer aid to seniors.

230
Macular Degeneration?

http://www.macd.net
As we age, our vision is typically impaired. Over 10 million Americans have macular degeneration. Be aware of what it is and what you can do about it.

231
Aging Gracefully

http://www.agingresearch.org
The Alliance for Aging Research is a private, not-for-profit advocacy organization fighting for science policies in the nation's capital, to speed breakthroughs for greater health, vitality and longevity.

232
A Kid at Heart

http://www.worldhealth.net
You have to visit a site that believes this: "The process of physical aging can be slowed, stopped or even reversed through existing medical and scientific interventions. We seek to bring about a profound shift in the way the medical field approaches human aging."

CHAPTER VIII
MEDIA AND MORE

233
It's the Real Thing

http://www.real.com
One of the most exciting technologies on the Internet is RealAudio. This allows you to listen to and sometimes watch broadcasts on the Net. Some of the sites below use this product. If you don't have it, you can get it (for free) at this site.

234
Family Health Radio

http://www.fhradio.org
Hosted by Ohio University, this site contains practical, easy-to-understand answers to some of the most frequently asked questions about health and health care. You'll also find a series of articles dating back to 1993.

235
NPR Health
http://www.npr.org/news/healthsci
"All things considered," this is an excellent source for high-quality, in-depth health information.

236
The Network
http://www.thehealthnetwork.com
Watch "TV" using RealAudio, and get information on every health topic.

237
Broadcasting Health and Fitness
http://www.broadcast.com/healthfitness
The folks who pioneered "radio" broadcasting on the Net offer lots of health and fitness content.

238
Let's Talk

http://www.healthtalkinteractive.com
This site labels itself as "real people connecting with experts for better health." You'll find specific networks that broadcast interviews and shows.

239
Body, Mind and Spirit

http://www.goddessradio.com
You'll find great interviews related to your body, mind and spirit.

240
Merck

http://www.merck.com
http://www.merck.com/pubs/mmanual/sections.htm
The world famous Merck manual is at this site. You'll also find quizzes and other interesting facts.

241
Physician's Desk Reference
http://www.pdr.net/consumer
This trusted name has a "getting well" section and many other news and information sources.

242
By the Way, Doctor
http://www.harvardhealthpubs.org
Harvard has health publications for a fee, but for free you can obtain its glossary and many questions and answers.

243
Medical Update
http://www.mdinteractive.com
http://www.1stheadlines.com/health1.htm
These interesting sites provide you with news feeds from some of the major medical and news Web sites.

244
Consumer Health Information
http://www.nih.gov/health/consumer/conicd.htm
The National Health Institute has online publications for almost every area of health. Go through the list, and take note of the areas that interest you.

245
FDA Magazine
http://www.fda.gov/fdac/fdacindex.html
Read some great articles from the Food and Drug Administration's magazine, FDA Consumer. It has articles from 1995 to the present.

246
Quality on Your Platter
http://webmedlit.silverplatter.com
http://webmedlit.silverplatter.com/sources.html
WebMedLit offers easy access to the best medical journals on the Web. It scans premier medical sites each day and extracts the available citations, abstracts and full-text articles.

247
American Council on Science and Health
http://www.acsh.org
These folks have many timely and informative articles. Scan to see which ones interest you.

248
Prevention
http://www.healthyideas.com
Prevention magazine has a Web site dedicated to providing healthy ideas.

249
Science Daily
http://www.sciencedaily.com/news/health_medicine.htm
Science Daily provides "your link to the latest health research news."

250
Health Online: Truth and Virtual Lies
http://www.msnbc.com/news/161811.asp
Here's an article that provides some hints, tips and clues on how to evaluate medical information that you find on the Net.

251
CNN Health
http://www.cnn.com/HEALTH
Current health news and all health subjects are covered.

252
Go To ABC
http://abcnews.go.com/sections/living
The ABC News site has a "health and living" section that has information from major publications.

253
CBS Health
http://www.cbs.com
At the CBS site, click on "Health" and you will get current news and information on the subject. You can even see a video version of the report.

254
Article From A to Z
http://www.wtvc.com/healthwatch/index.html
WTVC from Chattanooga has written health stories from "ADD" to "Zinc Lozenges." See if they have covered a story that would interest you.

255
Yahoo! Health News
http://dailynews.yahoo.com/headlines/health
Yahoo! has a daily health news section. Of course, there are other good health-related tidbits too.

256
Nutrition and Health News

http://www.wheatfoods.org/nutrnews.htm
The Wheat Foods Council has a section at its Web site with many articles from different publications. The articles are brief and informative.

257
My Health Magazine

http://www.zinezone.com
Go to the Zinezone and create your own health magazine. Just type "health" in the search box and you're on your way to having a great publication.

258
My News Page

http://www.newspage.com
The slogan here is "Knowledge is Power." NewsPage allows you to customize the news and information you receive, and health is one of the major categories.

259
Publishers Online
http://www.ncbi.nlm.nih.gov/PubMed/fulltext.html
This is a list of the journals for which publishers have provided links to their Web sites. Check it out to see if there is a publication you need to read.

260
Reuters Health
http://www.reutershealth.com
Reuters offers timely and detailed health information and articles.

261
Complete Medical Guide
http://cpmcnet.columbia.edu/texts/guide
Columbia University offers this medical guide (book) for free. Thirty-four chapters of information can make you a knowledgeable healthcare consumer.

262
Locate It Here

http://www.nlm.nih.gov/locatorplus
Do you need to find a book or an article about a specific medical issue? Search for it at this site.

263
Be Vibrant

http://www.vibrantlife.com
Here's a magazine for healthful living. Each month, you'll have interesting articles to read.

264
Men's Health

http://www.menshealth.com
The online version of this monthly magazine has current articles and archives of past articles for you to read.

265
Physician's Weekly
http://www.physiciansweekly.com
Get your weekly dose of highlights and analysis of medical news.

266
How's Your Health?
http://newsweek.com/nw-srv/focus/he/front.htm
"We've made great progress over the past 100 years, but a new poll suggests we're not as fit as we think." Let Newsweek explain why.

267
Weather and Health
http://www.weather.com/health
Allergy sufferers can find the pollen counts for their cities here. In-depth information on allergies, fitness, nutrition, drug information and much more is also available.

268
CNN and Allergies
http://www.cnn.com/WEATHER/allergy
On the Net, CNN can assist you with your allergies.

269
US News Health Reporter
http://www.usnews.com/usnews/nycu/health/hehome.htm
From health news to a health toolbox, you'll find lots of good stuff from U.S. News and World Report.

270
Best Hospitals
http://www.usnews.com/usnews/nycu/health/hosptl/tophosp.htm
U.S. News and World Report rates the best hospitals. If you have to go to the hospital, you might as well go to the best.

271
Health Index
http://usatoday.com/life/health/lhindex.htm
Here's an index to all the health stories written in USA Today.

272
Men's Health
http://www.nytimes.com/library/national/science/menshealth
The New York Times has current articles and a guide to more than twenty health topics.

273
Your Health
http://www.yourhealthdaily.com
More daily news and information about various health issues is available at this site that is also sponsored by the New York Times.

274
Medical Breakthroughs

http://www.ivanhoe.com
Using RealAudio, Ivanhoe Broadcasting will keep you current on some interesting breakthroughs.

275
The New England Journal of Medicine Says...

http://www.nejm.org
This oft-quoted journal is available online. Got a medical issue? Search for articles at this site.

276
Brits Journal

http://www.bmj.com
The British Medical Journal has a great Web site that has complete articles and archives.

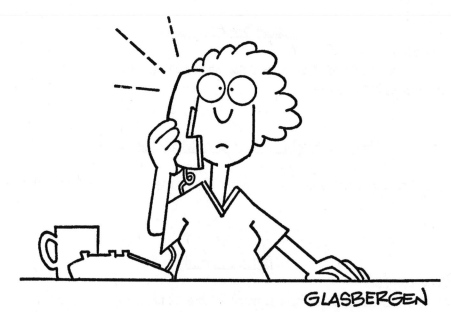

"Thank you for calling the Weight Loss Hotline.
If you'd like to lose 1/2 pound right now,
press 1 eighteen thousand times."

277
Med-News

http://www.incinc.net
Med-Brief covers important and timely research and medical news in a concise manner.

278
News Directory

http://www.healthnewsdirectory.com
Obtain current news and information on most health-related topics.

279
Magazine Stand

http://www.enews.com
Want to know what magazines are available on the subject of health? Enews will tell you. Just go to the "Health and Fitness" category.

280
Buy the Book

http://www.wellnessbooks.com
At this well-organized site, you can browse for books by category—from "Aids" to "Ulcerative Colitis."

281
Read On

http://www.medbookstore.com
It claims to be the "World's Largest Medical Bookstore." With over 90,000 books, the claim could be accurate.

282
Healthy Books

http://www.how2doit.net/HB.htm
Here's a site that has health-related books for sale. Read about them here and decide if any are for you.

283
PRNewswire
http://www.prnewswire.com/health/newshealthcare.html
Here are news releases from a wide range of companies, institutions, government agencies and other sources of health and biotech information.

284
The Lighter Side
http://www.medexplorer.com/humor/humor.dbm
A good attitude and sense of humor go a long way toward maintaining good health. You'll find humor, quotations, unusual statistics and other wit and wisdom here.

285
Ask Questions
http://ask.com/channels/health/fit.asp
AskJeeves.com is a fun and informative site. Ask any question, and you will be directed to many fine resources on the Net. And if you're curious, you can view some of the questions other people have been asking.

286
Health Search
http://www.isleuth.com/heal.html
The Internet Sleuth has over 20 health-related search engines at its site.
You are bound to find some good information here.

287
About Health
http://home.about.com/health
http://familymedicine.about.com
These sites will lead you to many fine health sites on the Net.

288
MicrosoftMD
http://health.msn.com
Microsoft is now doling out medical advice. In conjunction with WebMD, this
site has many timely health topics for you.

289
Yahoo! I'm Healthy

http://health.yahoo.com

The well-known search directory has a healthy amount of information. You can do searches for health topics or drugs and medications.

290
LycosMD

http://www.lycos.com/health

Join a community or a choose a topic in the "Focus on Health" area.

291
Medical Surf

http://www.medsurf.com

From "breakthroughs" to "recreation," you'll find many interesting and useful sites here.

292
Martindale's Health Guide
http://www-sci.lib.uci.edu/HSG/Medical.html
This is a virtual medical center that addresses almost every medical and health topic.

293
Librarian's Health Index
http://sunsite.berkeley.edu/InternetIndex/2/health.html
This librarian has categorized health topics ranging from "acupuncture" to "women's health."

294
Health Directories
http://www.healthlinks.net
http://www.healthwave.com
These sites are formatted in the style that Yahoo! has made famous. You'll find most of the major health categories covered here.

295
Search Profusion

http://health.profusion.com
Got a health question or issue? Profusion will search up to six health-oriented sites for you.

296
Stay Informed

http://www.medguide.net
This site states, "The best way to stay healthy is to stay informed." Use this medical search engine to accomplish that goal.

297
Doc and Patient Guide

http://www.pslgroup.com/docguide.htm
The goal of this site is to make it easier for doctors to use the vast resources of the Internet. There is a patient area as well. Check out the many resources available to you.

298
HMOs

http://www.4hmos.com
http://www.usnews.com/usnews/nycu/health/hetophmo.htm
Love 'em or hate 'em, they are here to stay. For timely information about HMOs, consult this site.

299
Select a Hospital

http://www.hospitalselect.com
http://neuro-www2.mgh.harvard.edu/hospitalwebusa.html
Select a hospital and get some detailed statistical information about it.

300
Direct Me to Health

http://www.hospitaldirectory.com
This site is more than just a hospital directory. Try out the life expectancy questionnaire or the health news directory for complete reporting on most healthcare topics.

INDEX (BY SITE NUMBER)

INDEX (BY SITE NUMBER)

INDEX (BY SITE NUMBER)

The Incredible Newsletter

If you are enjoying this book, you can also arrange to receive a steady stream of more "incredible Internet things," delivered directly to your e-mail address.

The Leebow Letter, Ken Leebow's weekly e-mail newsletter, provides new sites, updates on existing ones and information about other happenings on the Internet.

For more details about *The Leebow Letter* and how to subscribe, visit us at:

WWW.300INCREDIBLE.COM